YOGA

FOR CONNECTING

MIND,
BODY,
AND SOUL

For all ages, sizes, and schedules

LANA WEDMORE, AMED BERMUDEZ,
and MICHELLE BOOTH

Virginia

Published in the United States by WriteLife Publishing
(An imprint of Boutique of Quality Books Publishing Company, Inc.)
www.writelife.com

Printed in the United States of America

978-1-60808-238-4 (p)
978-1-60808-239-1 (e)

Library of Congress Control Number: 2020943558

Book design by Robin Krauss
Cover design by Rebecca Lown, www.rebeccalowndesign.com

TABLE OF CONTENTS

Shoulder and Upper Body Sequence

Neck Sequence

Balancing and Synchronizing the Hemispheres of the Brain

Bed Sequence

Airplane Sequence

Forest Bathing and Earthing

INTRODUCTION

I was waiting for two new guests to arrive at my eco-wellness lodge, Luna Lodge, on the Osa Peninsula in Costa Rica one summer afternoon. As I heard their car coming up the last hill, I walked over to the top of the stone driveway to greet them. One guest climbed out of the vehicle with ease but the other had more difficulty. She carefully maneuvered her way out with two canes—one in each hand.

I welcomed both guests with a glass of water and smiled as I escorted them, with caution, under the thatched roof of the Rancho Grande. We stopped for a moment as I showed them our world map covered with pins that represent the homelands of the fascinating guests who have traveled to Luna Lodge from 138 different countries.

Luna Lodge is located in a mountainous area in the middle of the rain forest. One can get around the property, but it is not for the weary or faint of heart. As the three of us continued walking, I thought to myself, *What am I going to do with this woman?*

My new guest had a beautiful face and it lit up when she heard the sounds of the howler monkeys nestled in the treetops around us. Seeing her radiate inner joy and light despite her physical limitations, I thought, *There is something under that skin that we can bring out and help her reconnect with.*

Nature is truly the best medicine. During her stay I performed a Shamanic Reiki session on her; my friend and soul mate, Amed Bermudez, gave her two massages; and I taught her some chair yoga. In four days we helped her ground back into Mother Earth and improve her gait. When it was time for her to leave, she walked down one of our beautiful slate paths—with a small declining slope—without any assistance. She wasn't using any canes and she was pulling her own suitcase. It was a miracle.

The key to being mentally alert, emotionally balanced, and positively inspired is to keep moving. We had helped my guest reconnect her mind, body, and soul in just a few days. She confided in me that she had only been living in her head for the past twenty years; she had totally forgotten about her body. It was at Luna Lodge where she remembered that the three truly are connected and they want to work together to make a better human being that has balance and harmony within. Our experience with that guest was the inspiration for this book.

I started doing yoga over thirty years ago. It has helped me spiritually, mentally, and physically, and I never could have built my Lodge without yoga in my life. Amed and I have been practicing, teaching, and doing yoga for the past fifteen years. Together, we have grown, helped, and supported each other on this path. We love teaching yoga to help people help themselves.

One does not write a book about a spiritual practice without practicing and experiencing some sort of inner results themselves. Yoga has added quality to our lives and we hope, to all of the people that we have taught. We wrote this book in service to others. One has to be eager and self-motivated to continue a practice but it is our hope that by teaching these yoga movements we can give people a gift that will serve and uplift them so they can see results and feel them even more.

We have watched as the world has become a sedentary society without movement. We need to get back to the basics. By that I mean basics of real living: sleep seven to eight hours a night without a phone under your pillow or even by your bed; drink seven to eight glasses of water a day; take at least ten minutes for yourself each day to meditate or move your body physically; and consider your eating habits. The key factor is not how much you eat, but the quality of the food you eat and how fast you eat it.

We need food and water to sustain life and our physical bodies, but more essential to us is the breath, the real food of life. They say that we are what we eat, but if you change the way you breathe you can change the person you are. Your mind follows the habits of the breath and the body so when you learn to control your breath you can control your mind. What a concept! Your health is the most important asset that you have and you are your own best doctor.

These pages were designed to help you start a daily ten-minute movement practice of your own. You will find breathing exercises, chair poses, and standing poses. We selected a variety of models to demonstrate the poses to show that people of all sizes, shapes, and ages can do them.

We took the photos outside at Luna Lodge because we live in the middle of the breathtaking rain forest in Costa Rica, but also to encourage you to get outside. You can do any of these poses indoors but, if you have the chance, do them out in nature.

We included a bed sequence in this book because I was traveling a lot and needed to do something before I got out of bed and started my day. We also added a sequence for an airplane flight. We all need to continue to move no matter where we are or what we are doing in our lives.

Your body loves you when you continue to listen to it and to give it love and attention. That is all anybody wants but, especially our own body. Listen to what it is trying to tell you. Become more aware of what life and nature are telling you.

With practice, you will find balance, become more comfortable, and connect with your own mind, body, and soul daily.

Peace within,
Lana Wedmore

LOWER BACK
SEQUENCE

PRAYER MUDRA

1. Sit comfortably in your chair, feet flat, spine straight.
2. Place your palms together.
3. Inhale and exhale deeply and smoothly through your nose.
4. Remain in this pose for 1 minute.

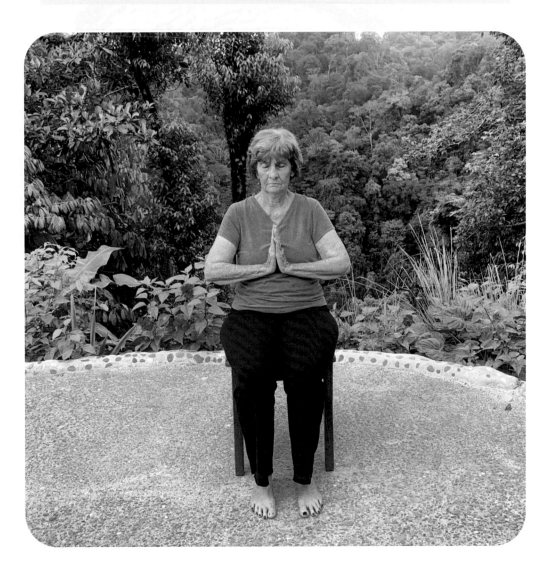

NECK AND UPPER BODY ROLL

1. Sit on the edge of your chair, feet flat, spine straight, hands on knees.
2. Move your upper body in big circles, keeping your neck relaxed.
3. Breathe deeply through your nose as you roll.
4. Roll in one direction for 30 seconds; then roll in the reverse direction for 30 seconds.

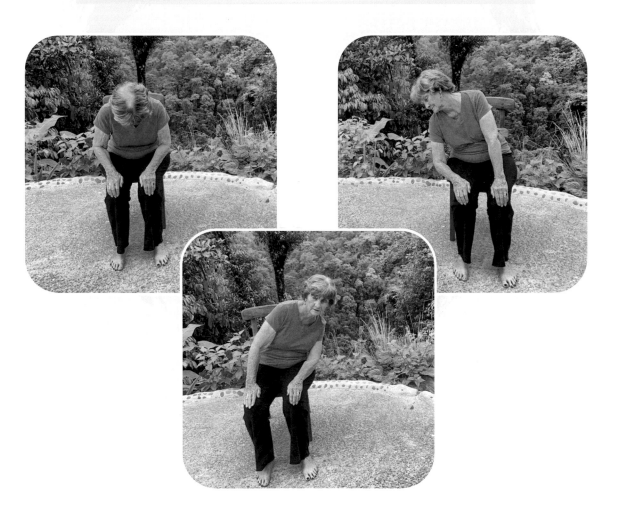

CAT AND COW

1. Sit on the edge of your chair, feet flat, spine straight.
2. Inhale as you flex the spine forward and lift the chest.
3. Exhale as you extend the spine backwards to round the back.
4. Keep breathing as you continue to flex and extend the spine for 1 minute.

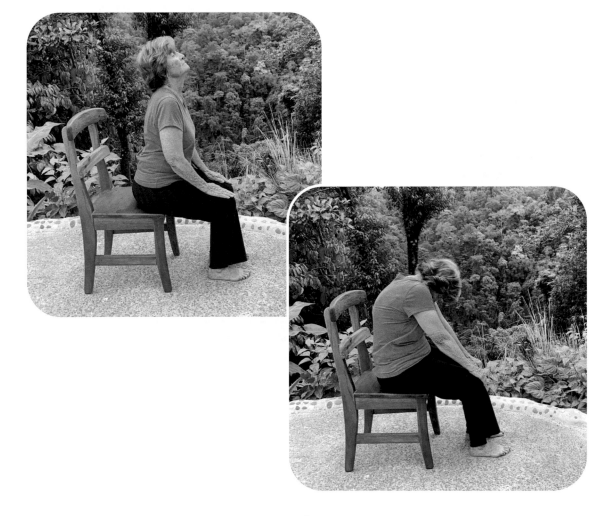

HIP OPENER

1. Sit on the edge of your chair, feet flat, spine straight.
2. Cross your right ankle over your left thigh just above the knee.
3. Flex your right foot.
4. Push the right knee down gently with your right hand.
5. Breathe deeply as you hold this pose and engage your core for 1 minute.
6. Continue breathing as you repeat this sequence with your left leg for 1 minute.

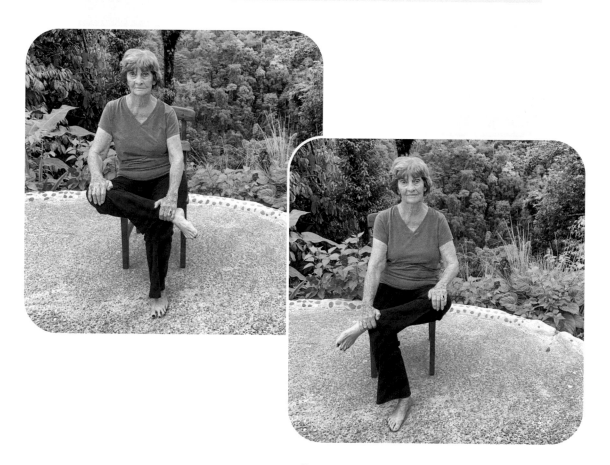

STRETCHING SIDE TO SIDE NECK ROLL

1. Sit comfortably on your chair, feet flat, spine straight.
2. Lift both arms and press your palms together.
3. Interlace your fingers and release the index fingers to point straight up.
4. Hold your chin away from your chest as you inhale, lifting your rib cage away from your hips.
5. Exhale for 3 breaths as you lean your upper body to the right, keeping your elbows straight.
6. Inhale for 3 breaths as you come back to center.
7. Exhale as you lean to your left side. Continue this sequence for 30 seconds.

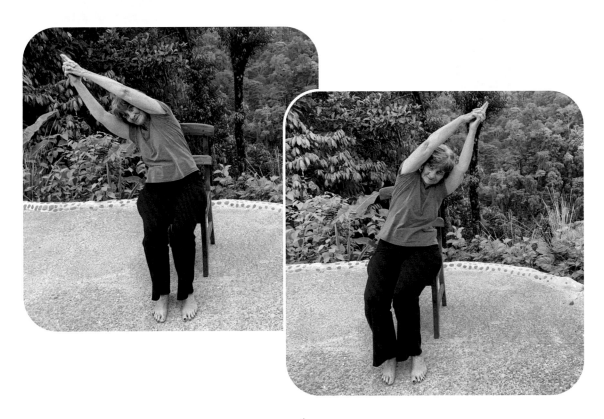

MEDITATION

1. Sit comfortably in your chair, feet flat, spine straight.
2. Hold your hands over your heart, feeling the beat.
3. Practice box breathing: breathe in through your nose, counting to 4 and hold the breath for 4 counts; breathe out through your nose for 4 counts and hold the breath out for 4 counts.
4. Continue box breathing for 1 minute.

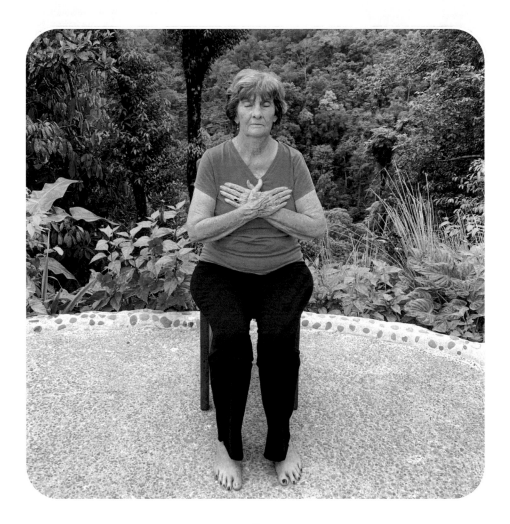

CORE TWIST SEQUENCE

MEDITATION

1. Sit comfortably in your chair, feet flat, spine straight.
2. Place your hands on your knees, palms facing up.
3. With each hand, touch your index finger to the pad of your thumb.
4. Breathe slowly, close your eyes, and focus on your breath for 1 minute.

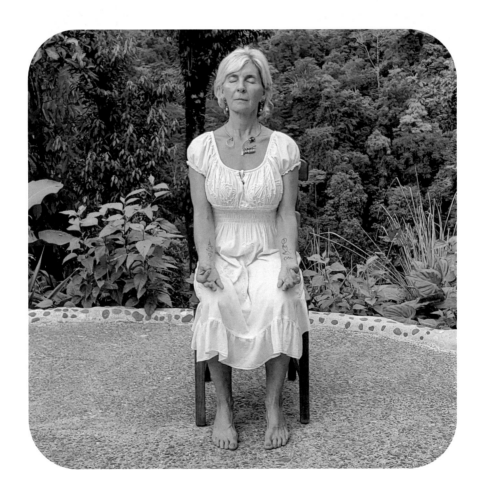

SINGLE-HAND CHAIR TWIST

1. Sit on the edge of your chair, feet flat, spine straight.
2. Inhale and twist to the right placing your left hand on the outside of your right knee and your right hand behind you on the back of the chair as you look over your right shoulder.
3. Breathe deeply for 1 minute.
4. Exhale as you let go and return to center.
5. Repeat on the left side, breathing deeply for 1 minute.

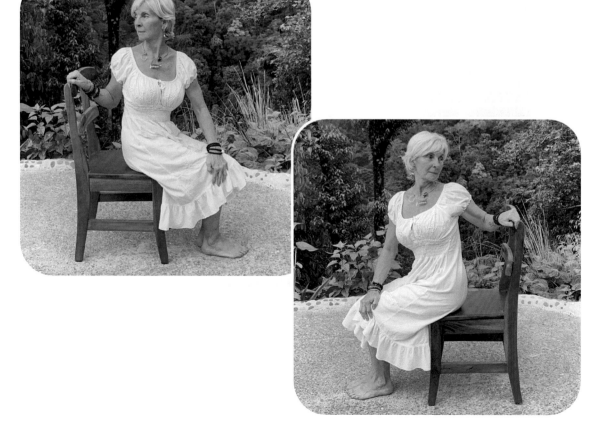

SPINAL TWIST

1. Sit on the edge of your chair, feet flat, spine straight.
2. Bring your hands to your shoulders.
3. Grasp your right shoulder with your right hand and left shoulder with your left hand, fingers in front, thumbs in back.
4. Inhale as you twist your spine to the left and exhale as you twist to the right.
5. Close your eyes and continue this sequence for 1 minute.

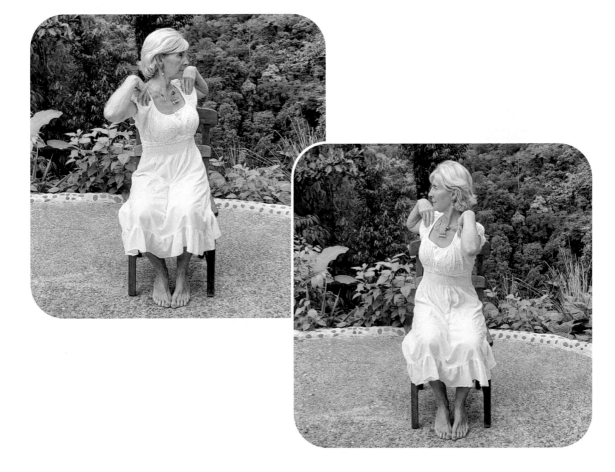

KNEE STRETCH

1. Sit on the edge of your chair, feet flat, spine straight.
2. Inhale as you interlace your fingers and clasp your right knee, gently pulling it close to your body.
3. Breathe deeply for 30 seconds.
4. Exhale as you gently release the pose.
5. Inhale and repeat on the left side, breathing deeply for 30 seconds.

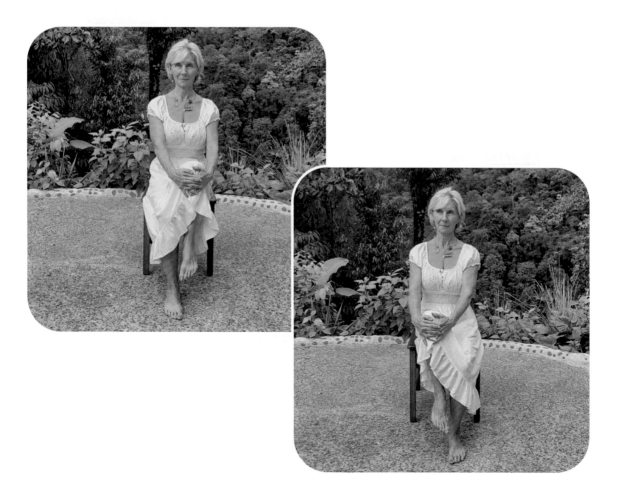

LEG KICKS

1. Stand in front of your chair, feet flat, hands on hips.
2. Find your balance. Gently kick your right leg forward and return to standing position.
3. Gently kick your left leg forward and return to standing position.
4. Continue this sequence for 1 minute, keeping your legs straight as you kick.

Variation: hold on to the back of the chair for balance.

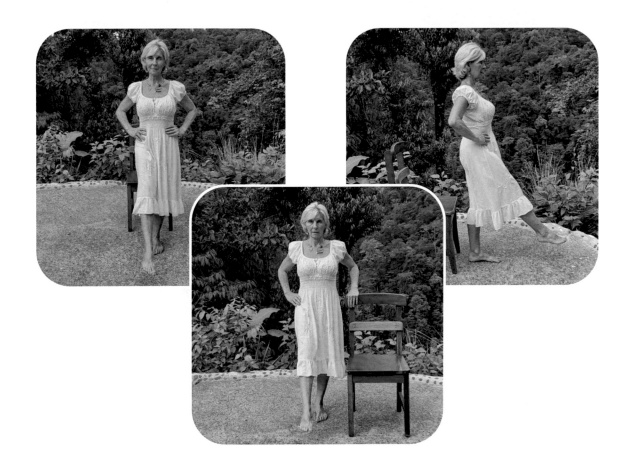

TWO-HAND CHAIR TWIST

1. Sit on your chair facing the right side, feet flat.
2. Inhale and twist to the right as you use both hands to grasp the back of the chair.
3. Breathe deeply for 1 minute.
4. Inhale as you release the pose and come back to center.
5. Repeat on the left side for 1 minute.

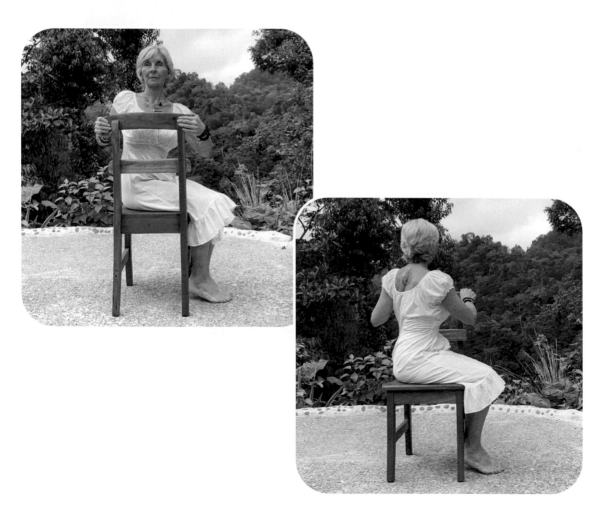

NECK STRETCH

1. Sit on your chair, feet flat, spine straight.
2. With your right hand, grab the seat of your chair; lift your left arm overhead placing your left hand over your right ear. Push gently as you stretch your neck to the left.
3. Breathe deeply for 30 seconds, then slowly release and come to center.
4. Inhale and repeat on the other side for 30 seconds.

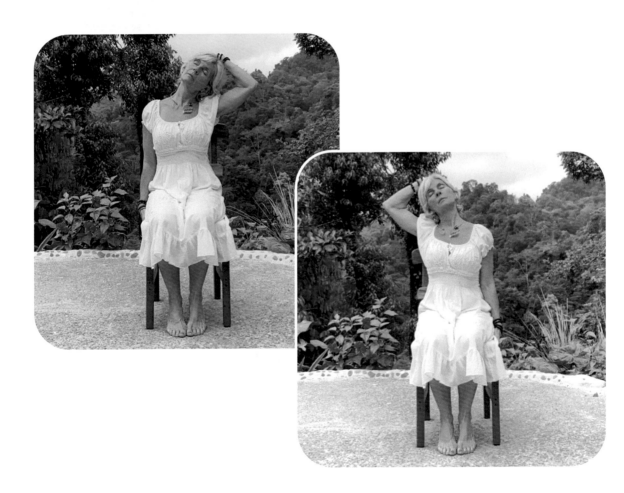

MEDITATION

1. Sit comfortably on your chair, feet flat, spine straight, eyes closed.
2. Place your hands in your lap, right palm under your left hand, thumb pads touching.
3. Breathe deeply for 1 minute, focusing on your breath.
   Go beyond time and space in total harmony and happiness.

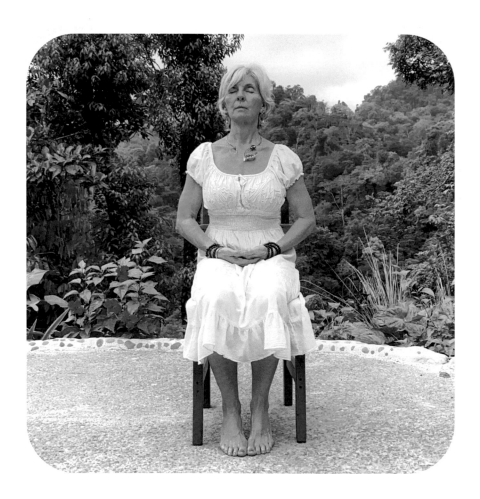

HEART — LUNG SEQUENCE

HEART MEDITATION

1. Sit on your chair, feet flat, spine straight.
2. Put your hands into a heart formation, over your heart.
3. Inhale and exhale as you meditate to the sound of your heartbeat.
4. Continue for 1 minute.

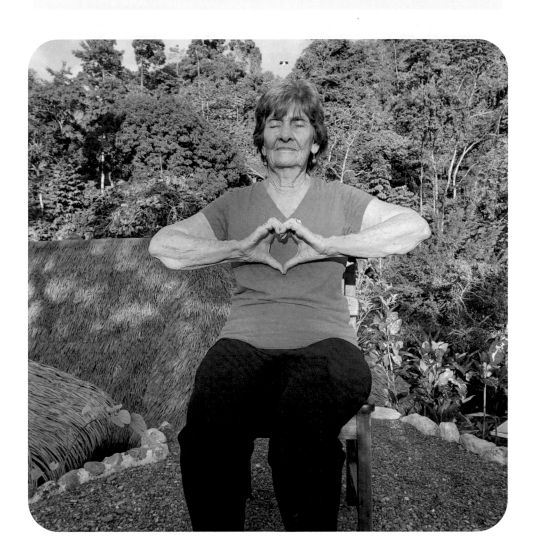

SEATED TWIST WITH ARMS EXTENDED

1. Sit on the edge of your chair, feet flat, spine straight.
2. Extend both arms out to each side and raise to shoulder height, parallel to the ground.
3. Curl your fingers into your palms with your thumbs pointing up.
4. Inhale as you twist your spine to the left and exhale as you twist to the right.
5. Continue this sequence for 1 minute.

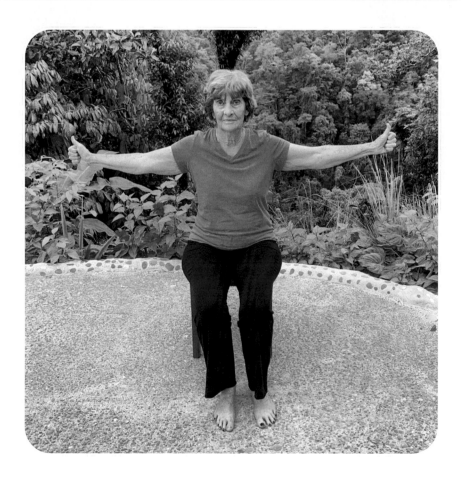

PENDULUM SHOULDER STRETCH

1. Sit on the edge of your chair, feet flat, spine straight.
2. Gently clasp your hands behind your back.
3. Lift your hands as you stretch your chest forward.
4. Inhale as you move your arms to the right and turn your head to the left.
5. Return to center and repeat on the opposite side.
6. Continue this sequence for 2 minutes as you focus on your breathing.

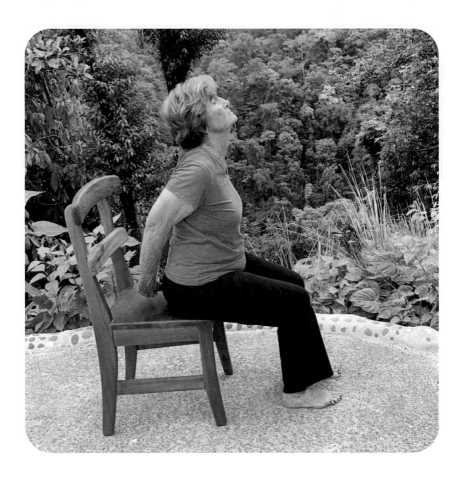

AIR PUNCHES

1. Sit on the edge of your chair, feet flat, spine straight.
2. Form fists with your hands and bring your arms close to your body, elbows bent.
3. Extend your left arm as you gently punch your left fist forward, keeping your right elbow bent, arm close to your side.
4. Begin alternating air punches.
5. Continue this sequence for 1 minute as you breathe deeply.

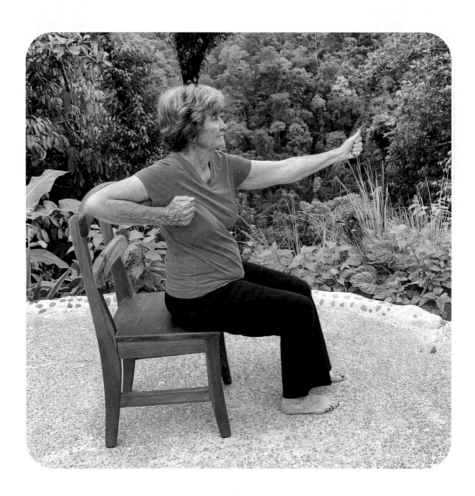

NECK STRETCH WITH HEAD TILT

1. Sit on the edge of your chair, feet flat, spine straight.
2. Interlace your fingers behind your neck and spread your elbows wide apart, pointing them up.
3. Inhale as you tilt your head back and look up.
4. Exhale as you tilt your head forward; relax your neck as you bring your chin to your chest.
5. Keep breathing as you bring your elbows down and bend forward.
6. Continue this sequence for 1 minute.

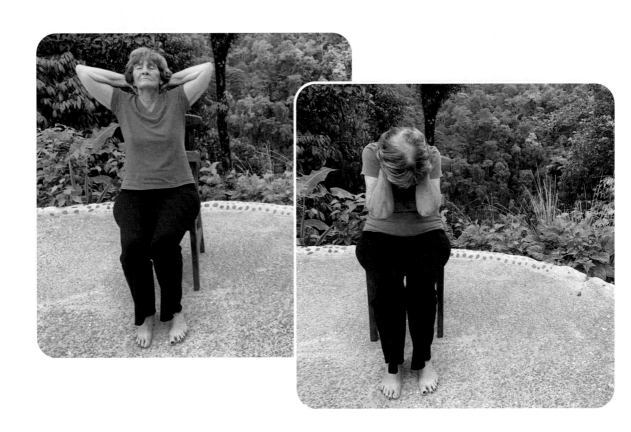

BEAR GRIP

1. Sit comfortably on your chair, feet flat, spine straight.
2. Interlock your hands at the heart-center of your chest, right palm facing down.
3. Hold your forearms parallel to the ground and your elbows out to each side.
4. Breathe deeply for 1 minute.

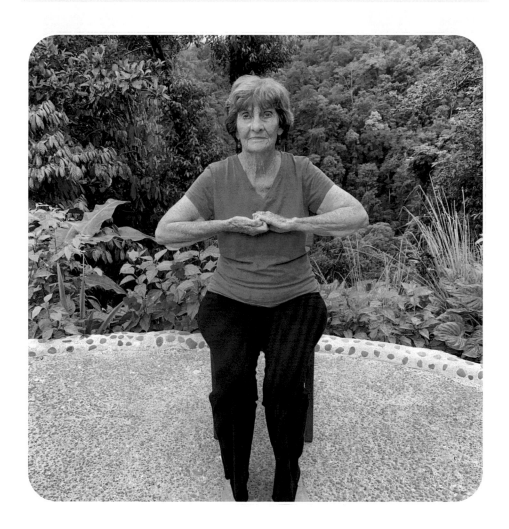

HEART MEDITATION

1. Sit comfortably on your chair, feet flat, spine straight.
2. Rub your palms together energetically, producing heat.
3. Bring your hands to your chest over your heart in prayer pose.
4. Concentrate on your heart-center; feel the connection.
5. Meditate and fill your heart with peace.
6. Continue breathing normally for 1 minute, or more if time allows.

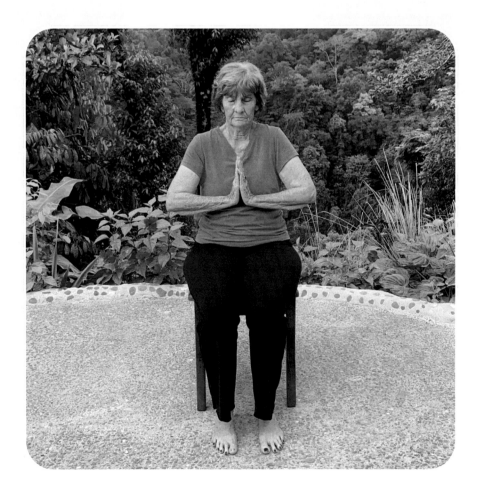

SHOULDER AND UPPER BODY SEQUENCE

MEDITATION

1. Sit comfortably in your chair, feet flat, spine straight.
2. Place your palms on your thighs.
3. Close your eyes and breathe deeply as you think positive thoughts for 1 minute.

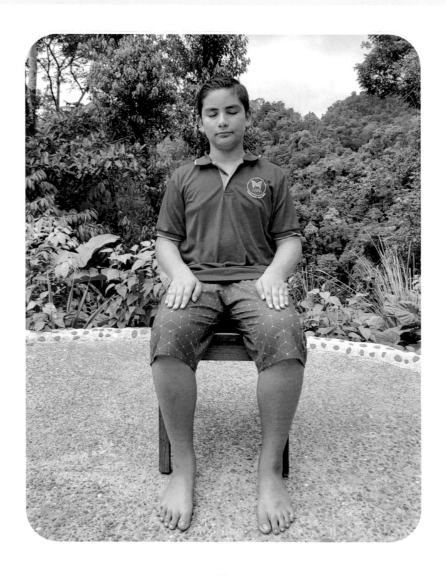

EAGLE ARMS

1. Sit comfortably on your chair, feet flat, spine straight. (You can also do this pose in the standing position.)
2. Inhale and stretch your arms up, palms facing each other.
3. Exhale as you wrap your right arm under your left arm and cross your elbows.
4. Cross your wrists so your palms touch (they will not overlap completely).
5. Lift both elbows to shoulder height and breathe deeply for 30 seconds.
6. Slowly release the pose.
7. Repeat with your left inner elbow under your right outer elbow, breathing deeply for 30 seconds.

Variation: cross your arms, placing each hand on the opposite shoulder.

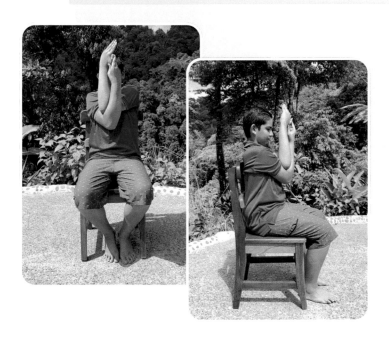
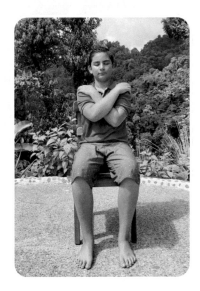

SHOULDER SHRUG

1. Sit comfortably in your chair, feet flat, spine straight, palms on your thighs.
2. Inhale as you lift your shoulders toward your ears.
3. Exhale as you drop your shoulders.
4. Continue this sequence as you breathe deeply for 1 minute.

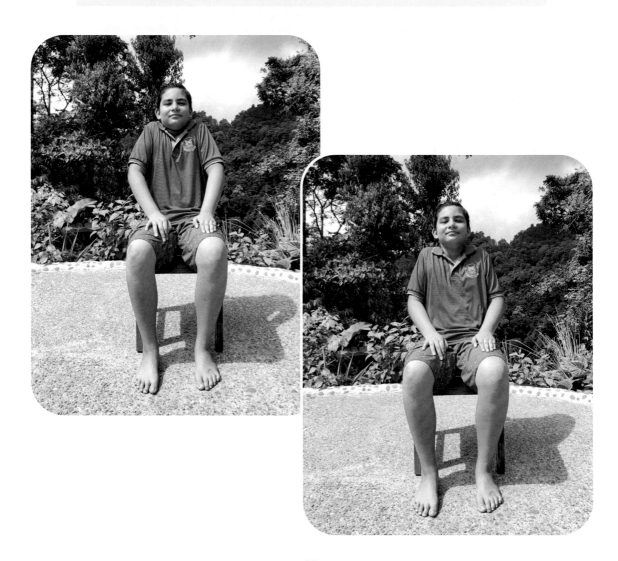

ROW THE BOAT

1. Sit comfortably in your chair, feet flat, spine straight.
2. Make fists with your hands and raise your arms to shoulder height, elbows bent at a 90-degree angle.
3. Breathe deeply as you rotate your shoulders and elbows forward for 30 seconds and row the boat.
4. Continue breathing deeply as you row backwards in your boat for 30 seconds.

Variation: row the boat in a standing position.

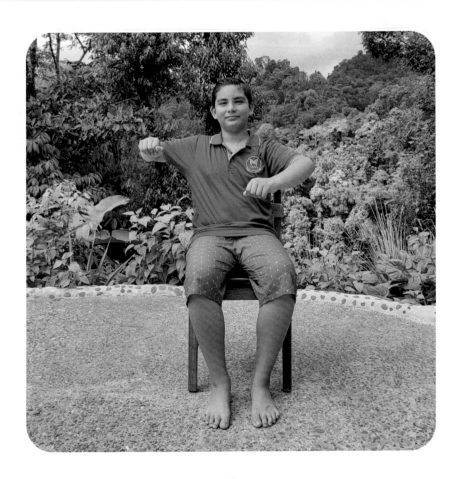

SHOULDER STRETCH

1. Sit in your chair comfortably, feet flat, spine straight. (You can also do this pose in the standing position.)
2. Stretch your arms overhead and bend your right arm, bringing your palm to the center of your upper back.
3. Place your left hand on your right elbow to gently stretch the right tricep.
4. Breathe as you hold this position for 30 seconds.
5. Release the pose and repeat on the opposite side as you breathe for 30 seconds.

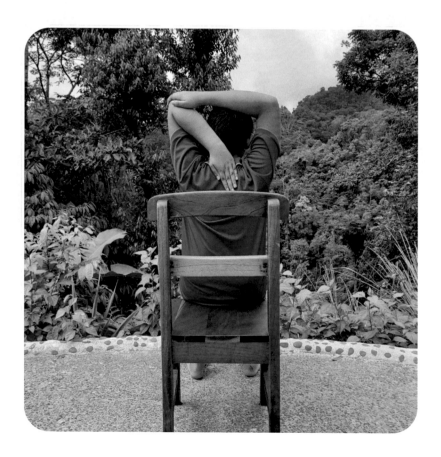

FOREARM AND WRIST STRETCH

1. Sit on the edge of your chair, feet flat, spine straight.
2. Place your forearms together and clasp your hands.
3. Breathe as you softly rotate your wrists in one direction for 30 seconds.
4. Continue breathing as you rotate your wrists in the opposite direction for 30 seconds.

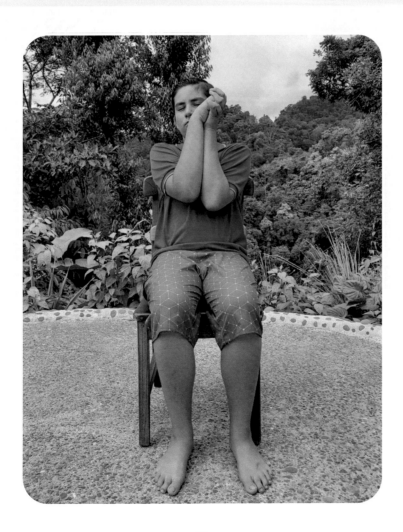

SHOULDER STRETCH WITH OPEN HEART

1. Stand in front of your chair, feet flat, spine straight.
2. Reach your hands behind you and clasp one hand in the other.
3. Inhale as you squeeze your shoulder blades together to open your heart.
4. Continue breathing as you gently lift your arms away from your body.
5. Exhale as you lower your arms.
6. Visualize releasing the tension in your upper body as you continue this sequence for 1 minute.

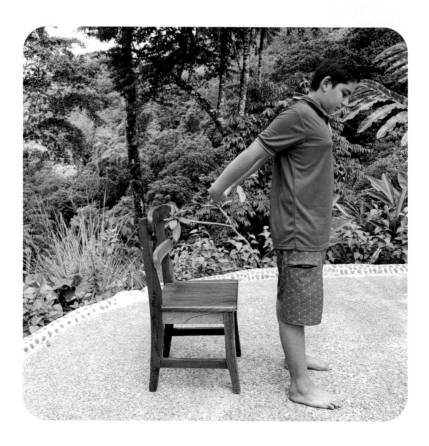

NECK STRETCH

1. Sit in a comfortable position in your chair, feet flat, spine straight.
2. Tilt your head back, chin lifted, and breathe deeply for 30 seconds.
3. Tilt your head forward, chin to chest, and breathe deeply for 30 seconds.
4. Come to center and breathe deeply for 1 minute.

Variation: alternate head tilt every 15 seconds.

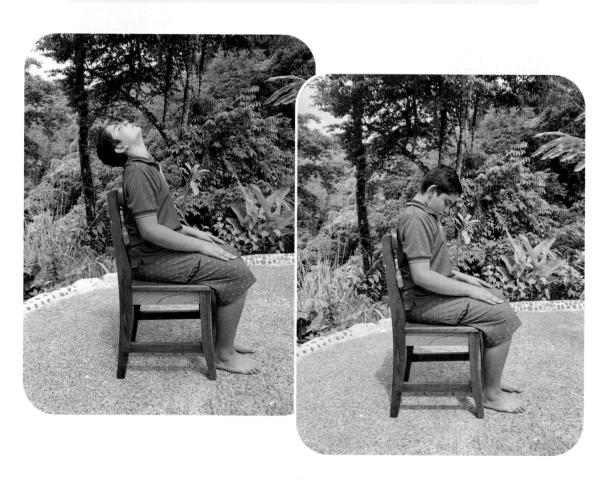

MEDITATION

1. Sit comfortably in your chair, feet flat, spine straight.
2. Put your hands in your lap, right palm on left, thumb pads touching.
3. Close your eyes and focus on your breath.
4. Continue breathing for 1 minute as you envision light shining on you and move into total harmony and happiness.

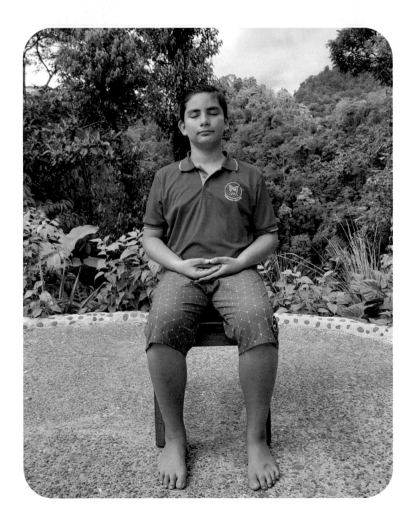

NECK SEQUENCE

ALTERNATE NOSTRIL BREATHING

1. Sit comfortably in your chair, feet flat, spine straight.
2. Place your right thumb on the right side of your nose and gently press the nostril closed.
3. Inhale and exhale slowly through the left nostril for 1 minute.
4. Release and repeat on the left side for 1 minute.
5. Release and breathe through both nostrils. Feel the energy flow through your body giving you health and life.

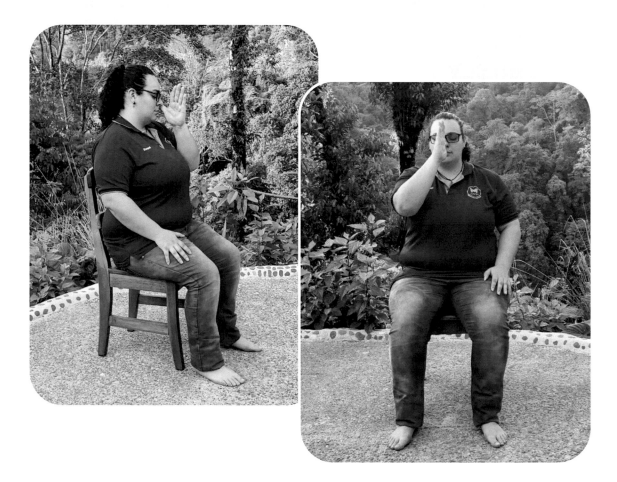

NECK ROTATION

1. Sit comfortably on your chair, feet flat, spine straight, palms on your thighs.
2. Inhale as you turn your head to the left.
3. Exhale and turn your head to the right.
4. Continue this sequence as you breathe for 1 minute.

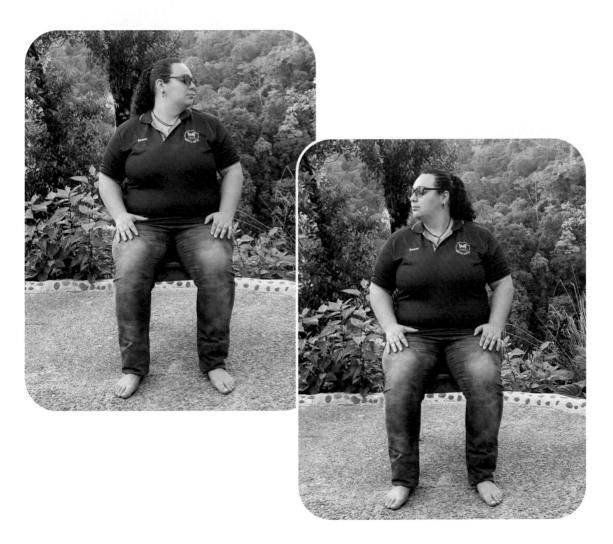

SMILING NECK

1. Sit comfortably on your chair, feet flat, spine straight.
2. Put a gentle smile on your face and look to the right.
3. Lower your chin to your chest and draw a smile across your chest as you rotate your head and neck to the left, and back to the right.
4. Continue drawing a smile from one side to the other for 1 minute while keeping a smile on your face.

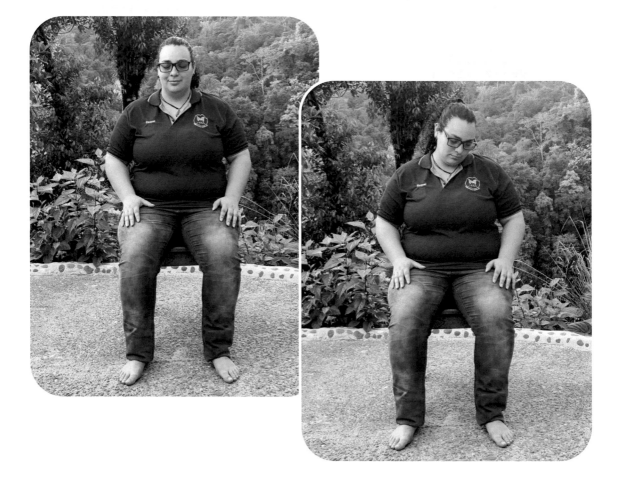

FIGURE-4 ARMS

1. Sit comfortably on your chair, feet flat, spine straight. (You can also do this pose in the standing position.)
2. Ground through your feet and reach your hands to the sky, palms facing each other.
3. Keep your right arm straight; bend your left arm to place your left palm on the outside of your right elbow.
4. Inhale as you raise your arms up.
5. Exhale as you lower your arms in front of you to the heart-center.
6. Continue to breathe as you raise and lower your figure-4 arms for 1 minute.
7. Release your arms and then repeat on the opposite side for 1 minute, keeping your left arm straight and placing your right palm on your left elbow.

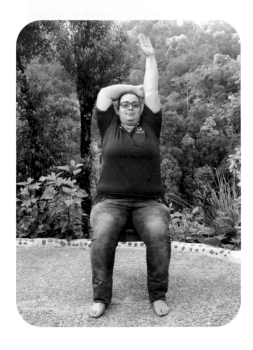 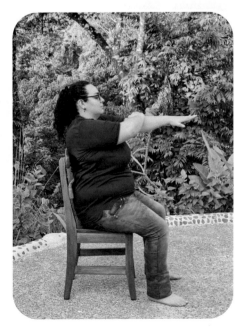

STANDING TWIST

1. Stand tall in front of your chair, feet hip-distance apart.
2. Cross your arms in front of you with your right forearm resting on top of your left forearm, palms on opposite elbows.
3. Inhale as you lift your arms overhead and twist to the left; exhale as you twist to the right.
4. Continue breathing as you twist for 30 seconds.
5. Release your arms and switch your grip.
6. Inhale as you lift your arms overhead. Breathe as you twist for 30 seconds.

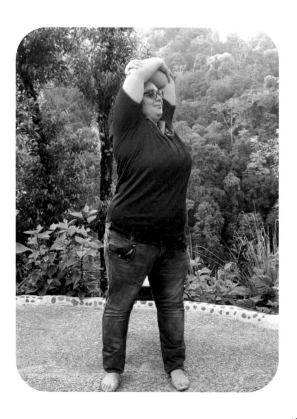
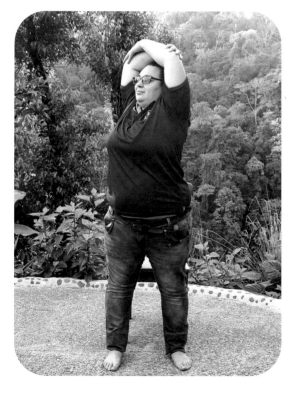

STANDING NECK STRETCH

1. Stand tall in front of your chair, feet hip-distance apart, engaging your core.
2. Assume prayer pose, placing your palms together, hands to your heart.
3. Inhale deeply as you stretch your arms, palms together, to a 60-degree angle and tilt your head back.
4. Exhale as you return your arms to prayer pose, bringing your head back to center.
5. Continue this sequence for 1 minute.

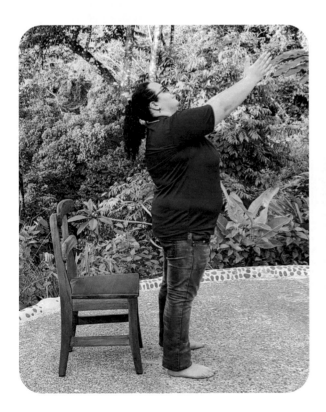
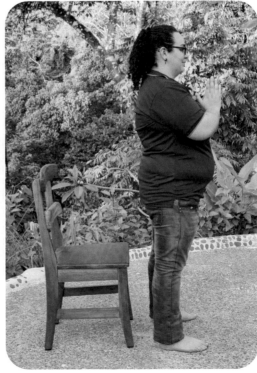

NECK SWIVEL WITH ARMS OUTSTRETCHED

1. Stand tall in front of your chair, feet hip-distance apart, engaging your core.
2. Raise your arms to shoulder height, palms facing up, parallel to the ground.
3. Inhale deeply as you swivel your head to the left.
4. Exhale deeply as you swivel your head to the right.
5. Continue this sequence for 1 minute.

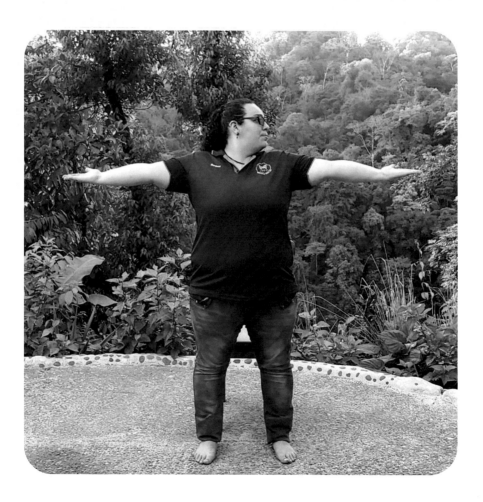

FACE YOGA

1. Sit comfortably on your chair, feet flat, spine straight.
2. Engage your core and place your palms on your thighs.
3. Breathe deeply as you make an "O" with your mouth and make the sounds "A" and "U."
4. Continue this sequence for 1 minute.

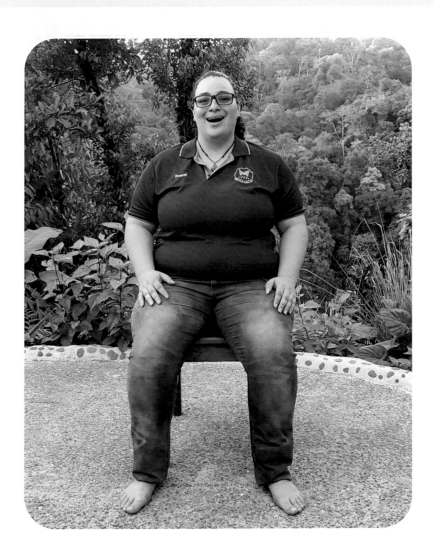

MEDITATION

1. Sit comfortably in your chair, feet flat, spine straight.
2. Interlock your fingers with your right index finger on top of the left; join your thumbs together and point them straight up.
3. Hold your hands in front of your heart and relax your elbows down.
4. Feel safe within yourself as you close your eyes and breathe through your nose with a steady breath.

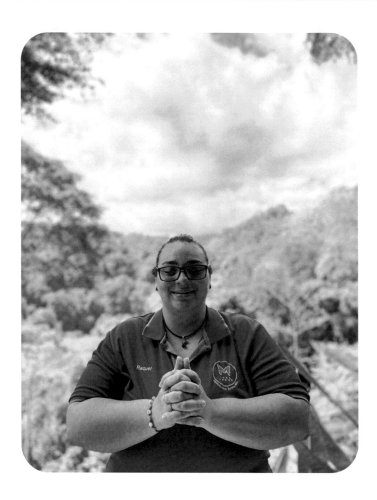

BALANCING
AND
SYNCHRONIZING
THE
HEMISPHERES
OF THE BRAIN

BREATH OF FIRE

1. Sit comfortably in your chair, feet flat, spine straight.
2. Breathe rapidly (2 to 3 breaths per second), like a panting dog.
3. Keep your breath continuous and powerful with no pause between the inhale and exhale.
4. As you exhale, push the breath out by pulling your navel and abdomen toward your spine.
5. Continue this sequence for 1 minute.

Note: the inhale will feel easier than the exhale because of the natural force of the diaphragm relaxing.

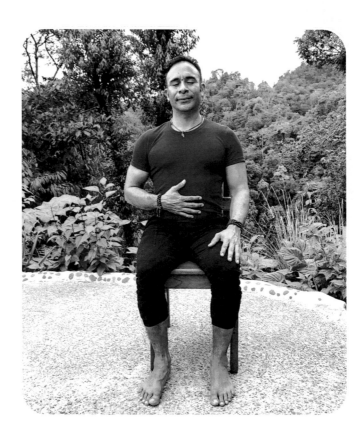

BALANCING THE HEMISPHERES OF THE BRAIN

1. Sit in your chair comfortably, feet flat, spine straight.
2. Make fists with your hands, tucking your thumbs inside.
3. Position your hands at heart level with your forearms parallel to the ground and elbows pointed out.
4. Without bending your wrists, rotate your fists rapidly around each other in circles, as you practice Breath of Fire.
5. Continue this sequence for 1 minute.

Variation: do not practice Breath of Fire.

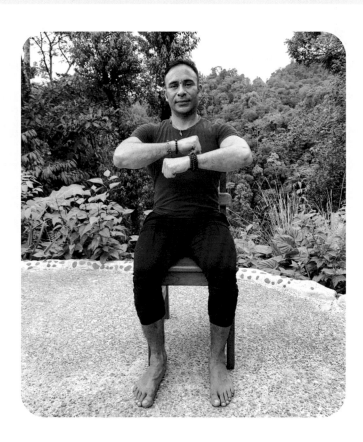

STAND STRAIGHT

(open circulation to the head)

1. Stand tall in front of your chair.
2. With your arms hanging down at your sides, form fists with your hands, tucking your thumbs inside.
3. Let your head fall back and gaze at a fixed point above you.
4. Hold this pose for 1 minute as you breathe slowly through your nose.

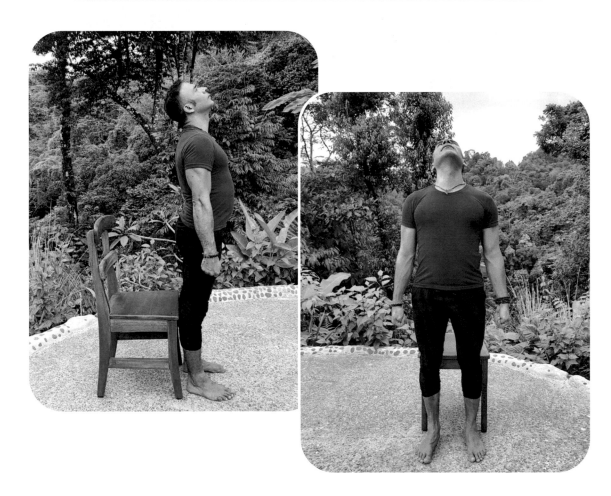

SPINAL FLEX

1. Sit on the edge of your chair, feet flat, spine straight.
2. Keep your head straight and shoulders relaxed, palms resting on your thighs.
3. Inhale and flex your upper body as far forward as you are able, sliding your palms to your hips and pushing your elbows back.
4. Exhale and round your back, sliding your palms over your knees and extending your arms straight.
5. Continue this sequence, breathing slowly for 1 minute.

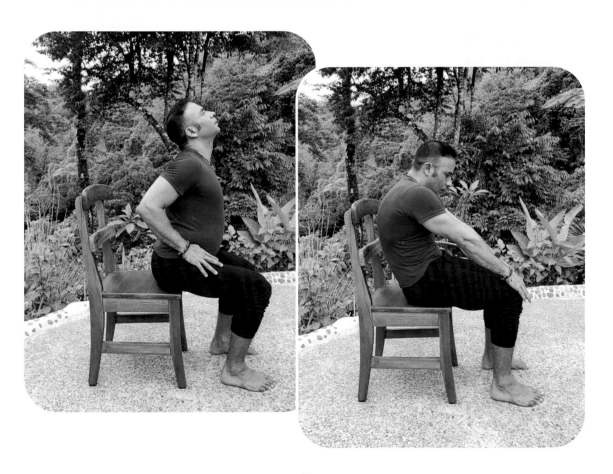

SPINAL TWIST

1. Sit on the edge of your chair, feet flat, spine straight.
2. Place your hands behind your neck and interlace your fingers, elbows pointing out.
3. Close your eyes and inhale as you rotate to the left.
4. Exhale and rotate to the right.
5. Continue this sequence for 1 minute.

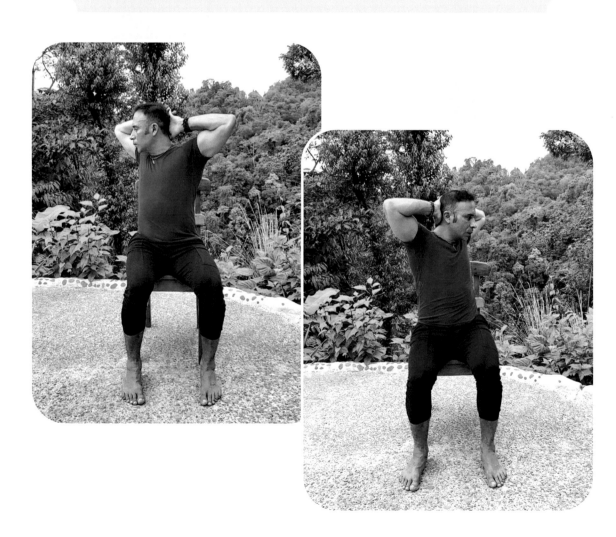

STANDING BEND WITH ARMS OVERHEAD

1. Stand in front of your chair, feet hip-distance apart.
2. Stretch your arms above your head, palms facing each other.
3. Inhale and bend to the left.
4. Exhale and bend to the right.
5. Continue this sequence for 1 minute.

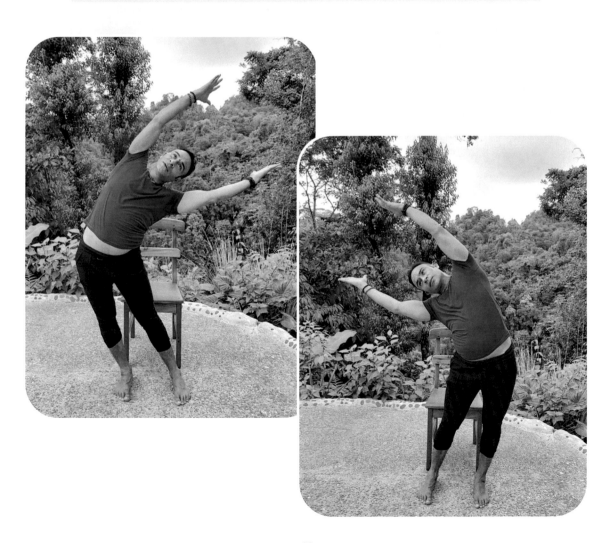

RUN ON THE SPOT

1. Stand in front of your chair, feet hip-distance apart.
2. Lift your left knee above hip-level while keeping your left arm tucked to your side and gently punching your right arm forward at shoulder level.
3. Switch sides, lifting your right knee and gently punching with your left arm.
4. Continue this sequence for 1 minute.

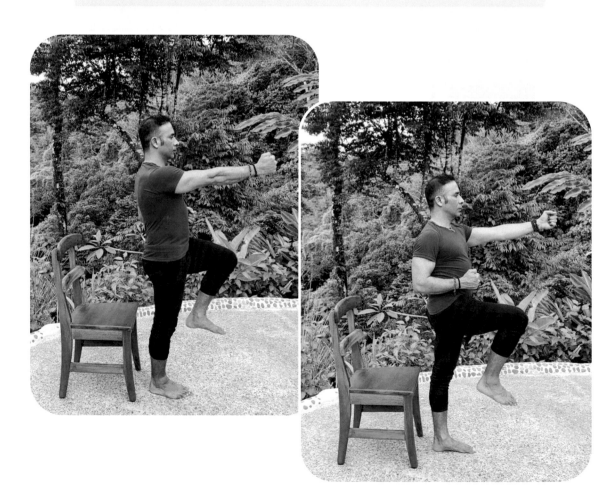

SIDE TO SIDE STRETCH

1. Sit on the edge of your chair, feet flat, spine straight.
2. Place your hands on your shoulders with the fingers in front and thumbs in back, elbows pointed out.
3. Inhale as you bend your upper body to the left; exhale and bend to the right.
4. Continue this sequence for 1 minute.

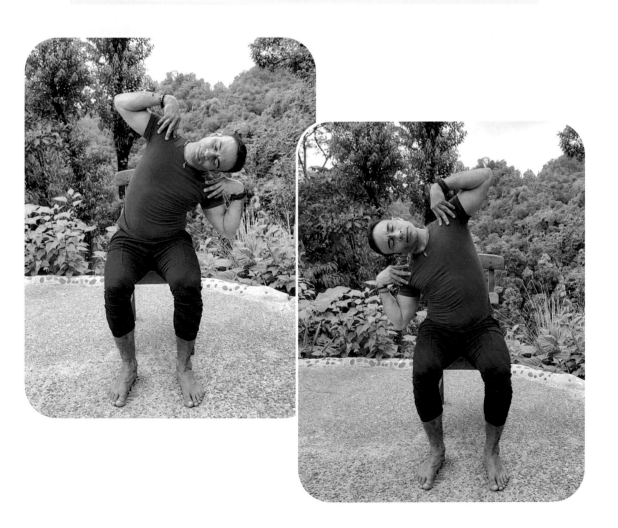

MEDITATION

1. Sit comfortably in your chair, feet flat, spine straight, chest lifted.
2. Lift your hands to chin level, fingertips together, pointing up to form a tent.
3. Close your eyes as you mentally chant a positive affirmation.
4. Breathe deeply for 2 minutes.

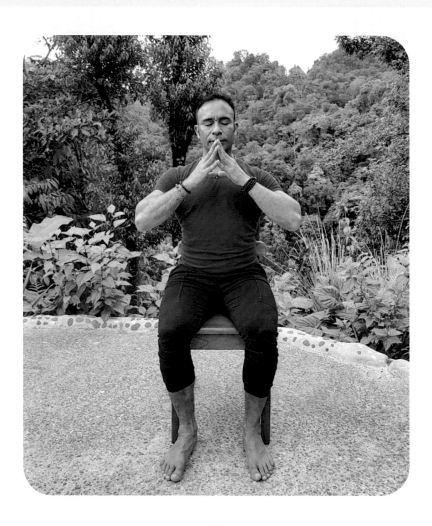

BED
SEQUENCE

THANKFUL MEDITATION

1. Lie face-up on your bed, arms alongside your body, palms facing up. (Corpse Pose or Shavasana)
2. Spread your legs apart and relax your whole body, including your face.
3. Gently bring a small smile to your face and close your eyes.
4. Inhale long, slow, and deep into the abdomen for 1 minute. As your abdomen expands and fills, allow your chest to rise and fully receive the complete breath.
5. Feel your abdomen expand on the inhale and contract on the exhale.
6. Roll over to your right side and continue breathing slowly.
7. Slowly rise up to a seated position.

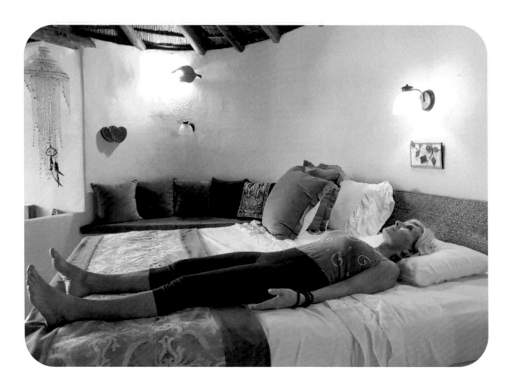

NECK ROLLS

1. Sit cross-legged on your bed, spine straight, palms on your knees.
2. Lower your chin to your chest and gently roll your head and neck in a circle to the right.
3. Continue for 30 seconds, breathing slowly and deeply, keeping the shoulders relaxed.
4. Repeat to the left for 30 seconds.

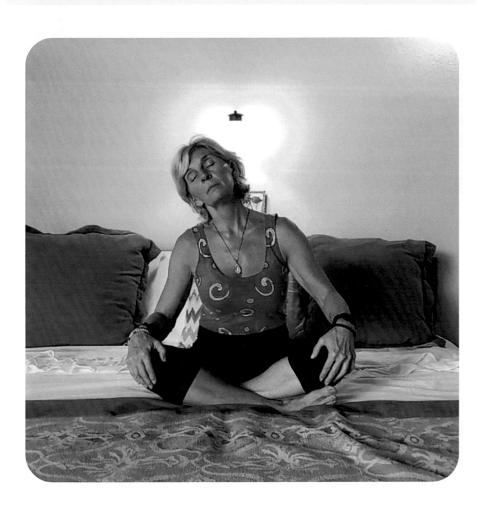

UPPER BODY ROTATION

1. Sit cross-legged on your bed, spine straight, palms on your knees.
2. Inhale slowly as you gently rotate your upper body in a circle to the right for 30 seconds, opening your hips.
3. Keep your neck relaxed and engage your core.
4. Come back to center, then rotate to the left for 30 seconds.

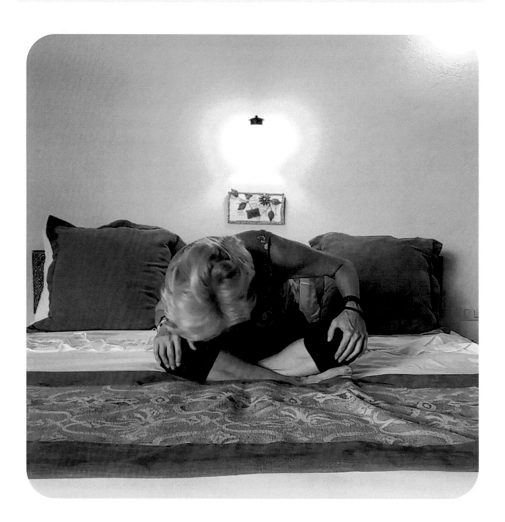

SPINAL FLEX (CAT AND COW)

1. Sit cross-legged on your bed, spine straight, palms on your knees.
2. Inhale as you press your chest forward and roll your shoulders away from your ears.
3. Exhale as you round your head, neck, and shoulders, pulling your navel to your spine and extending your spine back.
4. Continue this sequence for 1 minute.

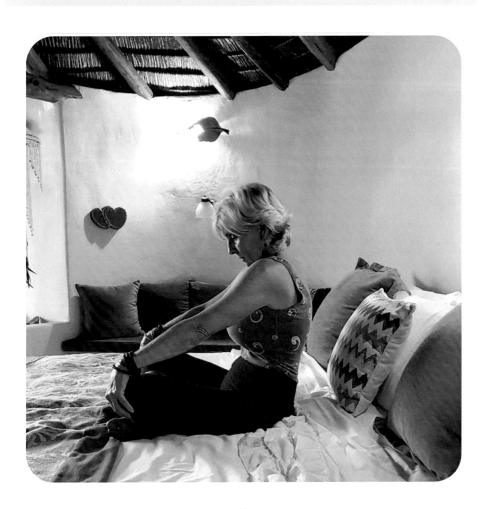

SPINAL TWIST

1. Sit cross-legged on your bed, spine straight.
2. Place your right hand on your left knee.
3. Position your left arm behind you, palm flat with fingers facing away from you.
4. Gently twist your upper body to the left and look over your shoulder.
5. Breathe deeply for 30 seconds.
6. Return to center, then twist to the right, breathing deeply for 30 seconds.

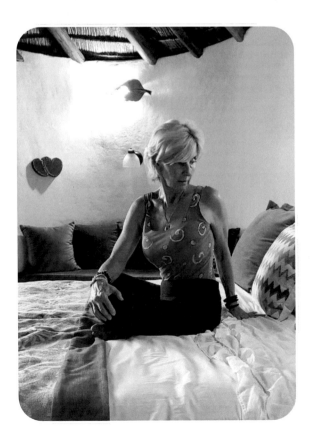
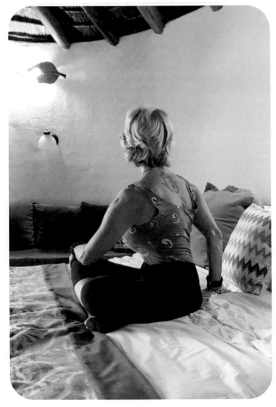

SIDE TO SIDE STRETCH WITH ARMS OVERHEAD

1. Sit cross-legged on your bed, spine straight.
2. Lift your arms overhead and interlace your fingers; release the index fingers to point straight up.
3. Lift your chest and drop your shoulders away from your ears.
4. Lift your chin away from your chest, keeping your elbows straight and your biceps in line with your ears.
5. Inhale as you lift your rib cage away from your hips, lengthening your body.
6. Exhale as you gently stretch your upper body to the right.
7. Keep your elbows straight, ears between your biceps, chin lifted.
8. Continue breathing as you hold this pose for 30 seconds.
9. Return to center, then repeat on the left side for 30 seconds.

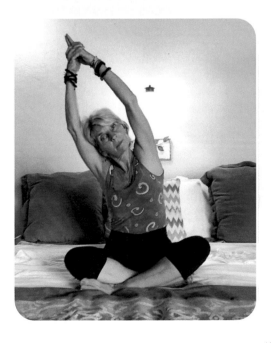 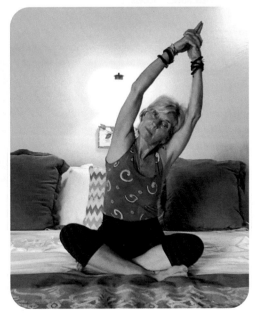

SPINAL TWIST WITH HANDS TO SHOULDERS

1. Sit cross-legged on your bed, spine straight.
2. Place your fingertips on top of your shoulders, fingers in front, thumbs in back.
3. Inhale as you gently twist your upper body to the left.
4. Exhale as you twist to the right.
5. Continue breathing as you repeat this sequence for 1 minute.

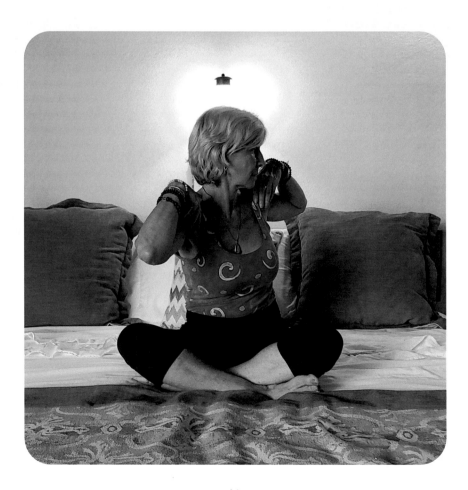

FORWARD BEND

1. Sit on your bed with your legs straight forward, spine straight.
2. Inhale as you lift your arms overhead.
3. Continue breathing as you lengthen up through your fingers and crown of your head, keeping your neck relaxed.
4. Exhale as you hinge forward at your hips.
5. Slowly lower your torso toward your legs and grab your toes.
6. Keep your spine erect and your toes flexed toward you.
7. Breathe normally for 1 minute.

Variation: rest your palms on your legs instead of grabbing your toes.

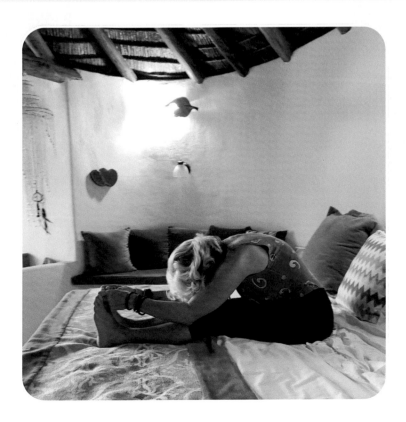

MEDITATION

1. Sit cross-legged on your bed, spine straight.
2. Bring your palms together in front of your heart and close your eyes.
3. Direct all your attention to your body and feel every single part of your body.
4. Breathe slowly for 1 minute, staying calm.

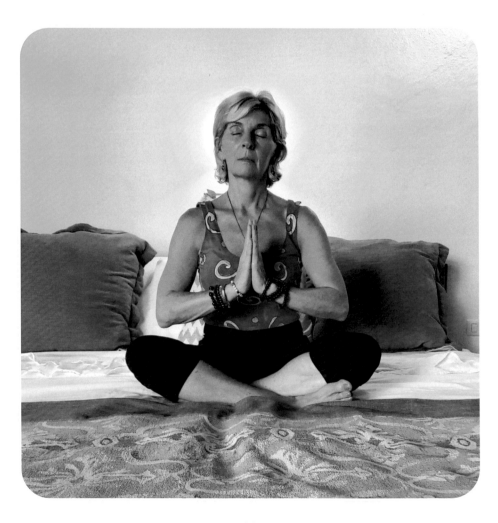

AIRPLANE SEQUENCE

MEDITATION

1. Sit comfortably in your seat, feet flat, spine straight.
2. Stretch your arms straight in front you at shoulder height.
3. Breathe deeply for 30 seconds.
4. Bring your palms together in front of your heart, breathing deeply for 30 seconds.
5. Focus on the flow of your breath.

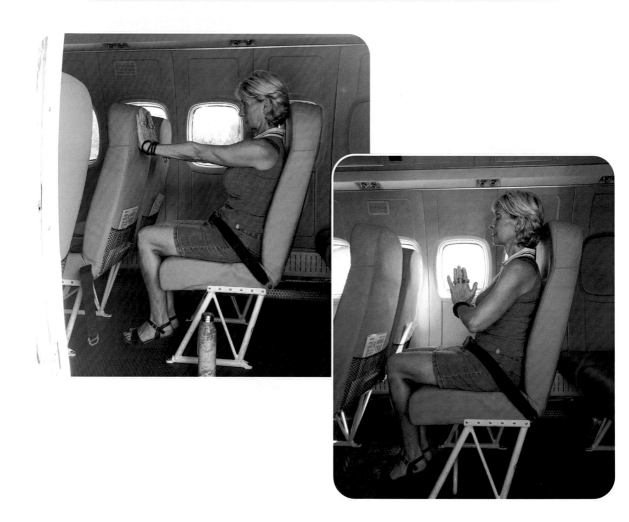

SPINAL FLEX

1. Sit comfortably in your seat, feet flat, spine straight, palms on knees.
2. Inhale as you draw your shoulder blades back and push your spine forward.
3. Exhale as you round your head, neck, and shoulders forward, pulling your navel to your spine and extending the spine back.
4. Continue breathing as you repeat this sequence for 1 minute.

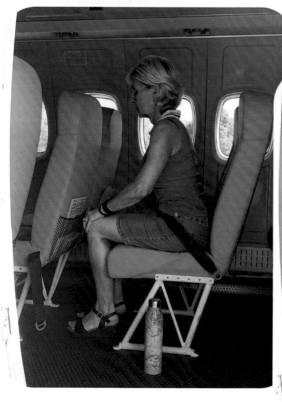
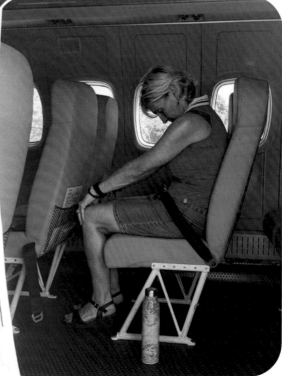

VENUS LOCK WITH ARMS OVERHEAD

1. Sit comfortably in your seat, feet flat, spine straight.
2. Press your palms together, interlace your fingers, and lift your arms overhead.
3. Rotate your wrists so your palms face up.
4. Breathe deeply for 30 seconds.

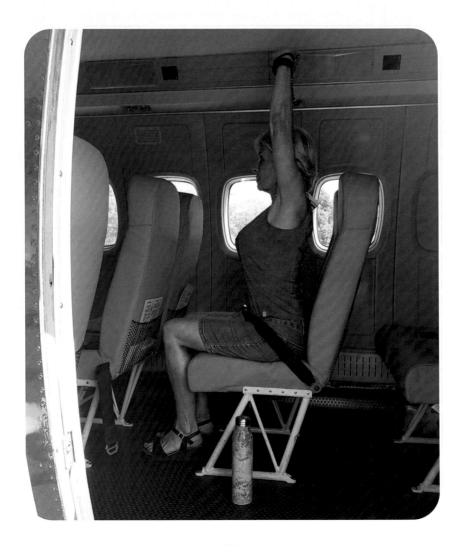

FOREARM AND WRIST TWIST

1. Sit comfortably in your seat, feet flat, spine straight.
2. Bring your forearms together in front of you at shoulder height and clasp your hands.
3. Breathe normally for 1 minute as you rotate your wrists and hands to the right.
4. Continue breathing as you rotate your wrists and hands to the left for 1 minute, noticing your mind calm as you do.

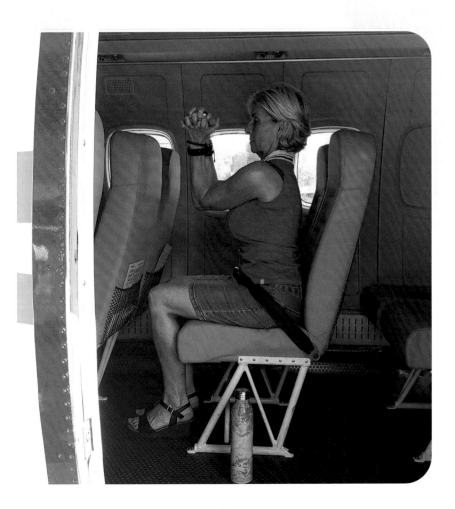

KNEE LIFTS

1. Sit comfortably in your seat, feet flat, spine straight.
2. Inhale as you clasp your left knee and draw it close to your body.
3. Breathe deeply for 30 seconds and then release your leg.
4. Repeat this sequence with your right knee, breathing deeply for 30 seconds.

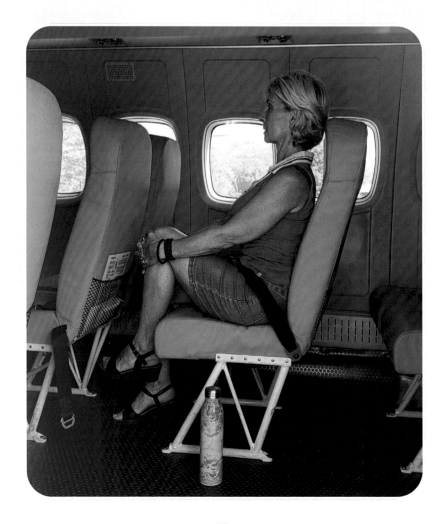

ARM RAISE WITH CLASPED ELBOWS

1. Sit comfortably in your seat, feet flat, spine straight.
2. Cross your forearms in front of you at shoulder height and grab your opposite elbows.
3. Inhale as you lift your arms overhead; exhale as you lower your arms back to shoulder height. Breathe normally as you continue this sequence for 1 minute.
4. Switch arms and repeat this sequence for 1 minute.

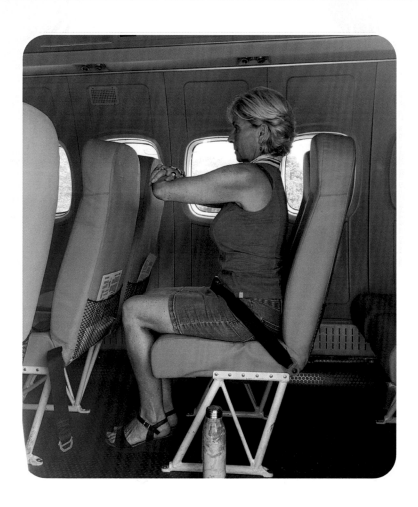

STANDING LEG LIFTS

1. Stand next to your seat, feet flat, spine straight, hands down at your sides.
2. Breathe normally as you straighten and lift your left leg forward.
3. Return to standing, then straighten and lift your right leg forward.
4. Continue this sequence for 1 minute.

Variation: hold on to your seat with one hand.

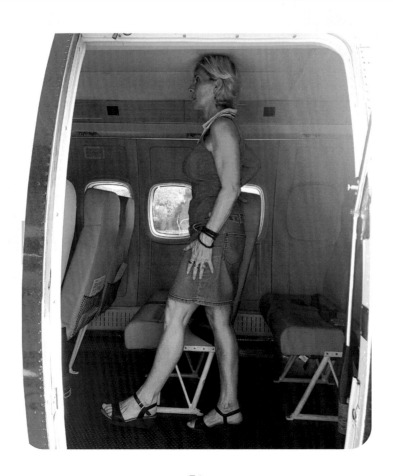

FORWARD BEND

1. Stand next to your seat, feet flat, spine straight.
2. Exhale as you hinge forward at your hips, leading with chest.
3. Bend your knees slightly as you fold halfway down, keeping your spine straight.

Get out of your seat and walk occasionally if you're able to do so.

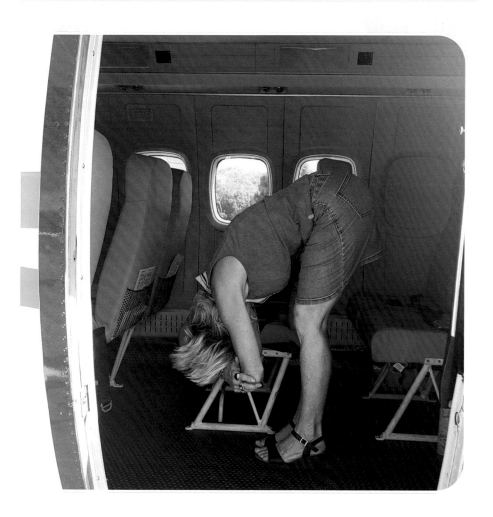

MEDITATION

1. Sit comfortably in your seat, feet flat, spine straight.
2. Bring your palms together in front of you at the center of your chest (prayer mudra).
3. Close your eyes and focus on your breath.
4. Breathe deeply for 1 minute, concentrating on the flow of your breath.

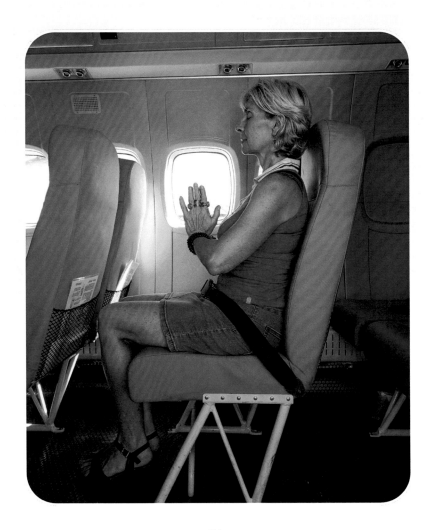

FOREST BATHING
AND
EARTHING

Connect to the earth.
Heal your body with the energy
of Mother Earth.

WALKING OUTSIDE IN NATURE

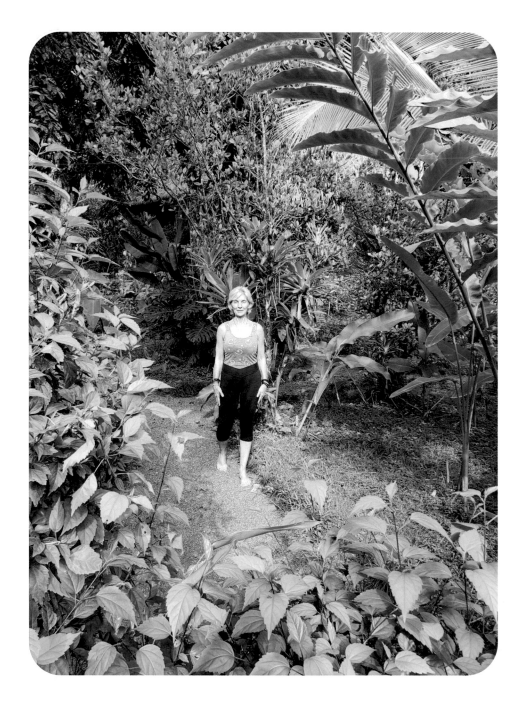

EARTHING WITHOUT SHOES

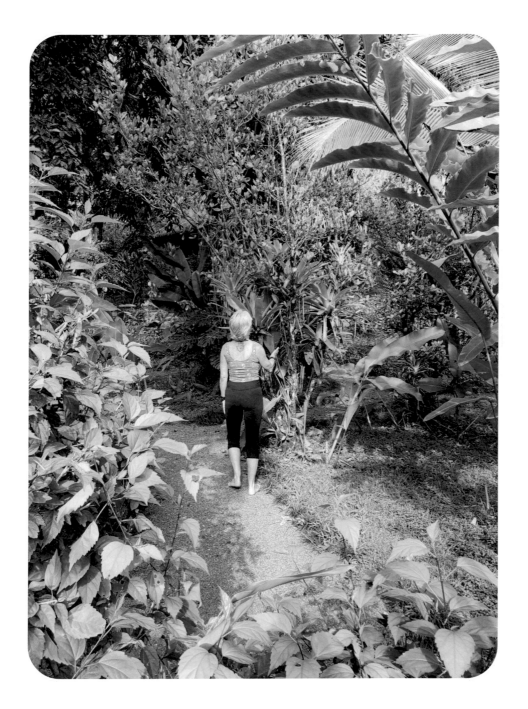

OBSERVING NATURE AND
ALL ITS WONDERS

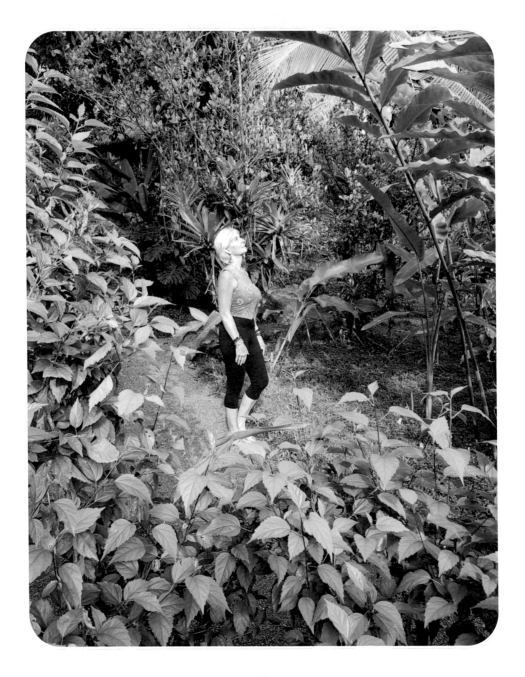

ACKNOWLEDGMENTS

First and foremost, we would like to express our sincere gratitude to Terri Leidich . . . thank you for suggesting we write this book, and for your continued support and advice throughout the publishing process.

Thank you to our models: Willie Ihrke, age 84; Raquel Alfaro Porras, age 28; and Erick Ahrat Ordoñez Fallas, age 12—all of whom agreed to demonstrate our ten-minute poses to illustrate that one's age, shape, or size should not discourage people from taking ten minutes a day to connect their mind, body, and soul.

The demonstrations for the Airplane Sequence were made possible by Skyway Airlines, Costa Rica. We appreciate your generous contribution.

Reiner Bravo Lopez helped us with the editing process for this book. Thank you for donating your time and expertise.

To all of you who are reading and using this book, we appreciate you for supporting us and allowing us to help you take charge of your own life and health. A healthy mind, body, and soul can transform you into a healthy human being and help make a healthy Mother Earth.

Thank you from our hearts and souls,
Lana and Amed

Life is not under your control and the mind is not obedient, but there is something the mind does obey. That is the rate of the breath. When the breath is long, deep, and slow, the mind is constant and calm.

ABOUT THE AUTHORS

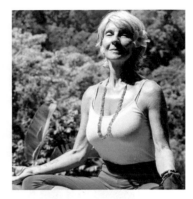

LANA WEDMORE is a registered, certified yoga instructor, and has been practicing and teaching yoga, pranayama, meditation, and philosophy for over thirty years. She is a certified Reiki master, a shamanic healer, a Certified Association of Nature and Forest Therapy (ANFT) forest therapy guide, and a trained sound-healing practitioner.

Nearly three decades ago, Lana built Luna Lodge, an innovative wellness eco-lodge on Costa Rica's Osa Peninsula. She facilitates empowerment retreats at Luna Lodge, speaks at prominent wellness and conservation events, and leads conservation initiatives for the White Hawk Foundation, which she founded in 2008 in the name of protecting the sacred land surrounding Corcovado National Park. Her mission is to "Heal within, help heal others, and heal Mother Earth."

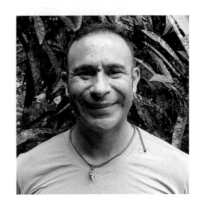

AMED BERMUDEZ is a registered yoga teacher and a Yoga Alliance certified education professional. He became a yoga instructor in 2005 and a massage therapist in 2007. He provides individual and group yoga instruction and individual massage techniques including deep tissue; hot stone; reflexology; gem therapy; Reiki; aromatherapy; tantra; and Shiatsu. With his shaman heritage, Amed offers a holistic approach to massage and yoga instruction. His belief is, "Your yoga practice is an opportunity to give yourself love and attention and become more aware of your body."

MICHELLE BOOTH has been helping people tell their stories for more than two decades. She ghostwrites autobiographies, memoirs, and family legacy books for a variety of clients including a former staff secretary in the White House Personnel Office. She also edits nonfiction manuscripts, and was selected to edit the memoir of a former NBA basketball player.

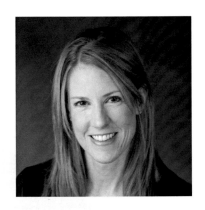

OTHER BOOKS BY LANA WEDMORE

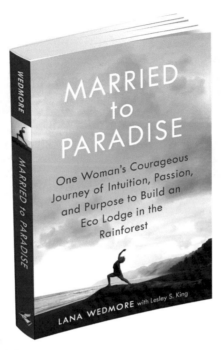

Forty years ago, a young Colorado ski racer falls in love with the freedom and sensuality of a remote Costa Rican rainforest. However, unlike most of us who return home from our tropical vacations, she sets out to make this sensation her life, and to help others experience it. With her own hands, and the help of a Costa Rican boyfriend, she builds an eco-lodge in the remote rainforest of Costa Rica's Osa Peninsula.

During her journey, a tractor trailer rolls over on her, breaking her leg in four places, her house burns to the ground, and she completely runs out of money. These calamities only strengthen her resolve.

In the end, she succeeds in building a lodge praised by media ranging from Travel + Leisure to CNN, and in helping people from all over the world experience one of the most biologically diverse places on earth. She also creates the nonprofit Whitehawk Foundation to save the Osa rainforest.

THE WHITE HAWK FOUNDATION

In 2008 Lana Wedmore founded The White Hawk Foundation in response to the growing urgency to protect the land surrounding Corcovado National Park. Educating people locally and internationally about conservation is a passion of Lana and her team of guides. Lana's message is very simple: "We must save the rain forests to save ourselves."

The White Hawk Foundation is a place where individuals and philanthropic entities can make a tangible difference. In the last ten years, contributions have enabled the foundation to acquire and protect land that could have been devastated by commercial or agricultural development. This land has been donated to a conservation easement, protecting it into perpetuity.

The mission of the White Hawk Foundation is to promote the preservation of the ecosystems and biodiversity of the Osa Peninsula in Costa Rica by engaging communities, research institutions, and businesses in a sustainable symbiotic relationship with nature.

You are welcome to make a donation or help spread the word. If you are a writer, reporter, or conservationist, please contact us to explore partnership opportunities. We would be grateful for the opportunity to work with you to protect one of the most bio-diverse places left on this planet.

Website: Whitehawkfoundation.org
Email: info@whitehawkfoundation.org
Call: 888.760.0760 (US and Canada) | 506.4070.0010 (Costa Rica)